Holistic Health for College Students

Practical Tips for Staying Healthy and Balanced in College

Angelina Sorenson

Holistic Health for College Students: Practical Tips for Staying Healthy and Balanced in College

Disclaimer

The information provided in this book is for educational and informational purposes only. While every effort has been made to ensure the accuracy and completeness of the content, the author/publisher makes no representations or warranties of any kind, express or implied, about the completeness, accuracy, reliability, suitability, or availability of the information contained herein.

The techniques, strategies, and suggestions presented in this book are based on the author's personal experiences and research. They may not be suitable for every individual or situation. Readers are advised to use their own discretion and judgment when applying any information from this book to their own circumstances.

The author/publisher shall not be held liable for any loss, injury, or damage arising from the use of the information contained in this book. Readers are solely responsible for their own actions and decisions.

Any references to specific products, services, or organizations are provided for informational purposes only and do not constitute an endorsement or recommendation. The author/publisher shall not be held liable for any consequences resulting from the use or misuse of such products, services, or organizations.

It is recommended that readers consult with qualified professionals or experts in the relevant field before making any significant decisions or taking any actions based on the information provided in this book.

By reading this book, the reader acknowledges and agrees to the terms of this disclaimer.

Dedication

For all the college students striving to find balance, health, and purpose amidst the whirlwind of campus life—this book is for you. May these pages offer you guidance, support, and a reminder to care for your well-being along the journey. To those who encouraged me and shared their insights, thank you for inspiring this work. Here's to a healthier, more fulfilling college experience for everyone.

Table of Content

Introduction: Navigating College Life and Prioritizing Health

Entering college marks the beginning of an exciting new chapter in your life, filled with opportunities for personal growth, academic challenges, and social adventures. Yet, as exhilarating as this journey can be, it often brings with it a unique set of challenges that can strain your physical, mental, and emotional well-being. Balancing the demands of coursework, extracurricular activities, and social life requires not only energy but also a solid foundation of health and wellness. Unfortunately, many students find themselves overwhelmed, leading to stress, burnout, and a decline in their overall quality of life.

In this fast-paced environment, it can be easy to neglect your health. Late-night study sessions, unhealthy eating habits, and irregular sleep patterns become the norm for many. The pressure to excel academically and socially can overshadow the importance of self-care. However, prioritizing your well-being is crucial for navigating the ups and downs of college life. By embracing a holistic approach to health, you can cultivate balance and resilience, equipping yourself to tackle the challenges that lie ahead.

This introduction sets the stage for understanding why a holistic perspective is essential for thriving in college. It invites you to explore the interconnectedness of mind, body, and spirit, and how nurturing each aspect can lead to a fulfilling and successful college experience.

The Unique Challenges and Opportunities of College Life

Stepping onto campus for the first time is an exhilarating experience filled with anticipation and excitement. The vibrant atmosphere, characterized by eager faces and the buzz of conversation, invites you to explore everything this new chapter has to offer. College is a transformative time marked by academic challenges, personal growth, and social connections. However, alongside this excitement lies the reality of significant stressors. Academic pressures, social dynamics, financial responsibilities, and the need for independence can weigh heavily on your shoulders. Balancing these various aspects while trying to maintain your health can feel daunting, making it essential to prioritize your well-being.

The unique challenges of college life can manifest in ways that jeopardize your health. As you navigate demanding coursework, long study sessions, and tight deadlines, you may find yourself sacrificing sleep and healthy eating habits. Late-night study sessions can easily turn into all-nighters, and convenience foods may become the norm. Meanwhile, the pressures to socialize and connect can lead to neglecting your mental well-being. Many students struggle with feelings of anxiety, depression, and burnout as they attempt to juggle the various demands of college life. Recognizing and addressing these challenges early is crucial for establishing a strong foundation for your college experience.

Why Health and Balance Are Essential for Success

Prioritizing health and balance is not just about avoiding illness; it's about enhancing your ability to succeed in college. Research consistently shows that students who maintain their well-being perform better academically and experience lower levels of stress. A balanced lifestyle supports your cognitive function, emotional resilience, and overall quality of life. When you invest in your physical and mental health, you equip yourself with the tools needed to face the challenges of college life head-on.

However, many students overlook their health amidst the chaos of college life. Late-night cramming, fast food meals, and irregular sleep patterns can lead to a cycle of poor health that ultimately impacts academic performance. Understanding the importance of self-care and balance is crucial for creating a fulfilling college experience. By nurturing your mind, body, and spirit, you can foster a sense of well-being that permeates every aspect of your life.

Overview of Holistic Health: Mind, Body, and Spirit

At its core, holistic health recognizes the interconnectedness of mind, body, and spirit. This approach emphasizes that true well-being encompasses more than just physical fitness; it involves nurturing all aspects of your life. A balanced lifestyle integrates proper nutrition, regular physical activity, mental clarity, emotional resilience, and social connections. By cultivating harmony among these elements, you empower yourself to thrive, even in the face of college challenges. This book embraces a holistic approach to health, offering practical tips and strategies that will guide you toward a healthier, more balanced college experience.

The holistic health perspective encourages you to view your health as a comprehensive system rather than isolated components. It recognizes that stress and anxiety can manifest physically, and poor nutrition can impact your emotional well-being. By addressing these factors collectively, you can create a foundation for a balanced lifestyle that supports your academic and personal goals. Throughout this book, you will learn to nurture each aspect of your well-being, recognizing that they are all interconnected.

How to Build Sustainable Habits for Wellness

Building sustainable habits is the key to maintaining your health throughout college. It is essential to recognize that change doesn't have to be drastic; small, incremental adjustments can lead to significant improvements over time. Instead of seeking quick fixes or trying to overhaul your entire routine, focus on making mindful choices that enhance your well-being. Start by incorporating more fruits and vegetables into your meals or setting aside just ten minutes each day for physical activity. The beauty of these changes is that they can fit seamlessly into your busy college life, allowing you to develop habits that become second nature.

This book serves as a roadmap for integrating holistic health into your college journey. Each chapter is designed to address a specific aspect of well-being, providing practical advice, relatable anecdotes, and actionable strategies. For example, you will learn about the importance of managing stress effectively, optimizing your sleep, and maintaining a nutritious diet—all essential components of a healthy lifestyle. Additionally, you'll discover the significance of prioritizing sleep and establishing a consistent sleep routine, significantly enhancing your ability to focus and retain information.

What This Book Offers to Help You Thrive During College

As you explore the chapters, you will find practical tips for managing stress and anxiety, which are common challenges for college students. Developing effective stress-relief techniques will enhance your resilience and adaptability in the face of academic pressures and social challenges. Furthermore, understanding the impact of nutrition on your cognitive function and emotional health will empower you to make informed choices about what you eat. You'll also learn about the importance of prioritizing sleep and establishing a consistent sleep routine, significantly enhancing your ability to focus and retain information.

One of the key themes throughout this book is the importance of self-care and self-compassion. College can be demanding, and it is easy to fall into the trap of perfectionism, pushing yourself to meet unrealistic expectations. Embracing self-care practices and treating yourself with kindness can help you maintain a healthy perspective on your journey. The book will encourage you to listen to your body and mind, recognizing when you need rest or support. Developing self-compassion can significantly reduce stress and anxiety, allowing you to thrive in both academic and social settings.

Building a supportive community is another essential aspect of your college experience. You don't have to navigate this journey alone; fostering connections with peers, mentors, and faculty can provide valuable support. The book will explore how to cultivate meaningful relationships and seek help when needed, as well as the importance of engaging with campus resources such as counseling services, wellness programs, and student organizations. Connecting with others who share your goals and values can be a powerful motivator for maintaining your health and well-being.

While the challenges of college life are real, the journey also offers immense opportunities for growth and self-discovery. As you navigate this period of transition, remember that your health is an ongoing journey, not a destination. The practices you establish now will not only benefit you during your time in college but will also lay the groundwork for a healthier, more balanced life beyond graduation. You have the power to shape your college experience, and prioritizing your well-being is the first step toward unlocking your full potential.

As you embark on this journey toward holistic health, keep in mind that change takes time and effort. Be patient with yourself and celebrate your progress, no matter how small. Embrace the knowledge that every step you take toward better health contributes to a more fulfilling college experience. With the right mindset and practical tools, you can cultivate a healthy, vibrant college life that prepares you for the future.

Welcome to *Holistic Health for College Students*! Within these pages, you will find the guidance and support you need to thrive during your college years. Let this book be your companion as you explore the principles of holistic health, learn to manage stress, cultivate resilience, and develop a balanced lifestyle. Your adventure toward a healthier, happier college experience begins here.

Chapter 1: Foundations of Holistic Health

As you embark on your college journey, understanding the foundations of holistic health is essential. In a world that often emphasizes academic achievement over personal well-being, it's crucial to shift your perspective to prioritize health in all its forms. Holistic health offers a comprehensive approach that integrates the mind, body, and spirit, recognizing that each component influences the others. This chapter will provide you with a foundational understanding of holistic health, its core principles, and how this approach can be beneficial as you navigate your college experience.

Many students arrive at college with preconceived notions about health, often viewing it through a narrow lens that focuses solely on physical fitness or the absence of illness. However, holistic health encompasses much more than that. It invites you to explore the connections between your mental state, physical well-being, and emotional resilience, creating a harmonious balance that fosters overall wellness. By the end of this chapter, you will be equipped with the knowledge to assess your health and set realistic goals for improvement, laying the groundwork for a successful and balanced college experience.

Defining Holistic Health and Its Core Principles

Holistic health is an integrative approach that considers the whole person—mind, body, and spirit—rather than focusing solely on individual symptoms or conditions. It emphasizes the importance of balance and harmony within these interconnected aspects of health, recognizing that neglecting one area can negatively impact the others. For example, chronic stress can lead to physical ailments like headaches or digestive issues, while poor nutrition can affect your mental clarity and emotional state.

The core principles of holistic health include:

1. **Interconnectedness:** Each aspect of health influences the others, and achieving balance requires attention to all areas—physical, mental, emotional, and spiritual.

2. **Individuality:** Recognizing that each person is unique, and what works for one individual may not work for another. Personalization is key in developing effective health strategies.

3. **Prevention:** Emphasizing the importance of preventive measures rather than solely treating existing health issues. This proactive approach encourages

individuals to make choices that promote long-term wellness.

4. **Empowerment:** Encouraging individuals to take an active role in their health journey, providing them with the knowledge and tools necessary to make informed decisions about their well-being.

Understanding these principles allows you to appreciate the importance of a holistic approach in your life. Rather than viewing health as a destination, consider it a lifelong journey that requires ongoing attention and effort.

The Interconnectedness of Mental, Physical, and Emotional Well-Being

One of the fundamental concepts in holistic health is the interconnectedness of mental, physical, and emotional well-being. Imagine your health as a three-legged stool: if one leg is weak or missing, the entire structure becomes unstable. Similarly, neglecting any aspect of your health can lead to imbalances that affect your overall well-being.

Mental Well-Being: Your mental state plays a crucial role in how you experience life. High levels of stress, anxiety, or depression can impact your academic performance and relationships. Practicing mindfulness, meditation, or engaging in activities that foster creativity can enhance your mental clarity and emotional resilience.

Physical Well-Being: Your physical health directly influences your energy levels and ability to focus. Regular exercise, nutritious eating, and adequate sleep are essential components of physical wellness. When you prioritize your physical health, you enhance your capacity to tackle academic challenges and enjoy social interactions.

Emotional Well-Being: Emotional health is often overlooked in the hustle and bustle of college life. Understanding your emotions and learning to cope with stress effectively can improve your overall well-being. Developing emotional intelligence—recognizing, understanding, and managing your feelings—allows you to navigate social dynamics and build healthy relationships.

Recognizing the interconnectedness of these areas is vital for creating a balanced lifestyle. Instead of addressing each aspect of health in isolation, aim for a comprehensive approach that considers how your mental state affects your physical health and vice versa.

How a Holistic Approach Can Benefit Students

Embracing a holistic approach to health can significantly benefit college students. The demands of academia, social life, and personal responsibilities can create a perfect storm for stress and burnout. By focusing on holistic health, you can enhance your resilience, improve your academic performance, and cultivate a greater sense of well-being.

Improved Academic Performance: When you prioritize your mental and physical health, you are more likely to perform well academically. Studies have shown that students who engage in regular physical activity and maintain a balanced diet tend to have better concentration, memory retention, and overall academic success.

Enhanced Stress Management: Holistic health encourages the development of effective coping strategies for managing stress. By practicing mindfulness, meditation, or yoga, you can cultivate a sense of calm and resilience, allowing you to navigate the pressures of college life more effectively.

Stronger Relationships: A holistic approach fosters emotional intelligence and self-awareness, which are crucial for building meaningful connections. As you learn to manage your emotions and communicate effectively, you can cultivate deeper, more supportive relationships with peers and faculty.

Greater Resilience: College life is full of challenges and unexpected events. A holistic approach equips you with the tools to adapt and bounce back from setbacks. By focusing on your overall well-being, you can build a strong foundation that helps you navigate obstacles with confidence.

Sustainable Health Practices: By understanding the principles of holistic health, you can develop sustainable habits that promote lifelong wellness. Instead of relying on quick fixes or fad diets, you'll be empowered to make informed choices that support your health journey.

Assessing Your Current Health and Well-Being

Before embarking on your journey toward holistic health, it's essential to assess your current health and well-being. This self-assessment will provide you with valuable insights into areas where you excel and areas that may need improvement. Take some time to reflect on the following questions:

Physical Health: Are you getting enough sleep? How often do you exercise? What does your diet look like? Do you have any chronic health issues that need attention?

Mental Health: How do you typically manage stress? Are you experiencing any symptoms of anxiety or depression?

How often do you take time for yourself to relax and recharge?

Emotional Health: Are you able to express your feelings effectively? How do you cope with challenging emotions? Do you have a strong support network to rely on?

Social Well-Being: How connected do you feel to your peers? Are you engaged in social activities that bring you joy? Do you have a sense of belonging on campus?

After reflecting on these questions, consider keeping a journal to track your thoughts and feelings over time. This process of self-reflection can help you gain clarity about your current state of health and identify specific areas for improvement.

Setting Realistic, Achievable Goals for Health Improvement

Once you've assessed your current health, it's time to set realistic and achievable goals for improvement. Goal-setting is a powerful tool that can motivate you to take actionable steps toward enhancing your well-being. When setting goals, keep the following guidelines in mind:

Be Specific: Instead of vague goals like "I want to be healthier," aim for specific objectives. For example, you might set a goal to exercise for 30 minutes three times a week or to incorporate one new vegetable into your meals each week.

Make It Measurable: Create measurable benchmarks to track your progress. This could involve keeping a food diary, recording your workouts, or using an app to monitor your sleep patterns.

Be Realistic: While it's important to challenge yourself, ensure that your goals are attainable within your current lifestyle. Setting overly ambitious goals can lead to frustration and burnout.

Time-Bound: Establish a timeframe for your goals. Whether you're aiming to achieve a goal by the end of the semester or within a specific month, having a deadline can increase accountability and motivation.

Celebrate Progress: Recognize and celebrate your achievements along the way, no matter how small. Positive reinforcement can boost your motivation and help you stay committed to your health journey.

By setting realistic goals, you can create a clear path for improvement and take proactive steps toward achieving your desired outcomes. Remember that change takes time, and it's essential to be patient with yourself throughout the process.

Chapter 2: Managing Stress and Building Resilience

Transitioning to college can be one of the most exciting yet stressful times in a young person's life. With newfound freedom comes an array of responsibilities and challenges, which can sometimes feel overwhelming. Understanding how to effectively manage stress and build resilience is crucial for navigating the complexities of college life. This chapter will delve into the common sources of stress that students encounter, offer practical techniques for daily stress relief, and explore the importance of resilience in fostering a balanced and healthy lifestyle.

As you journey through college, you'll likely face various stressors, from academic pressures and financial concerns to social dynamics and personal expectations. Learning how to recognize these stressors and develop strategies to manage them can empower you to maintain a sense of control and well-being. By building resilience, you can transform challenges into opportunities for growth, allowing you to thrive during your college years.

Understanding Common Sources of College Stress

College life is often a whirlwind of new experiences, responsibilities, and challenges. Understanding the common sources of stress can help you identify what may be affecting your mental and emotional well-being. Academic demands are a significant contributor to stress for many students. The pressure to excel in classes, meet deadlines, and prepare for exams can be daunting, particularly for those balancing multiple courses or extracurricular activities. As you strive for academic success, it is vital to recognize how these pressures can accumulate and impact your overall health.

Social relationships also play a critical role in the stress experienced by college students. Adjusting to new social environments can be intimidating. The desire to fit in, make friends, and navigate complex social dynamics can lead to anxiety and self-doubt. Furthermore, for many students, maintaining relationships with family and friends from home while trying to establish new connections can add another layer of emotional strain.

Financial pressures are another common source of stress for college students. Many individuals face significant student loans, tuition fees, and living expenses, leading to anxiety about future financial stability. Balancing work with academic responsibilities can also create tension, leaving little time for self-care or leisure activities.

Additionally, personal expectations can contribute to stress. Many students set high standards for themselves, whether in academics, social life, or personal achievements. When these expectations are not met, feelings of inadequacy or failure can arise, perpetuating a cycle of stress and self-criticism.

Practical Stress-Relief Techniques for Daily Use

Developing practical stress-relief techniques is essential for maintaining your well-being throughout your college journey. One effective method is mindfulness, which involves focusing your attention on the present moment without judgment. By incorporating mindfulness practices into your daily routine, you can reduce feelings of stress and anxiety while enhancing your overall sense of calm. Consider setting aside a few minutes each day for mindfulness meditation, deep breathing exercises, or simply taking a moment to appreciate your surroundings. These practices can help ground you, providing clarity and perspective amidst the chaos of college life.

Physical activity is another powerful tool for managing stress. Engaging in regular exercise has been shown to reduce symptoms of anxiety and depression while boosting overall mood. Whether it's going for a run, participating in a group fitness class, or simply taking a walk around campus, finding ways to incorporate movement into your routine can have profound effects on your mental health. Exercise releases endorphins, which are natural mood lifters, making it an excellent way to combat stress.

Establishing a balanced schedule is also crucial for stress management. Time management skills are essential for navigating academic demands while allowing time for self-care and relaxation. Consider creating a daily or weekly planner to organize your tasks and prioritize responsibilities. Breaking down larger assignments into smaller, manageable steps can help alleviate feelings of overwhelm and create a sense of accomplishment as you check tasks off your list.

Another technique to consider is journaling. Writing down your thoughts and feelings can provide an outlet for self-expression and reflection. Journaling allows you to process emotions, clarify your thoughts, and gain insight into the sources of your stress. It can also serve as a space for gratitude, where you acknowledge the positive aspects of your life, promoting a more balanced perspective.

Lastly, incorporating relaxation techniques such as yoga or progressive muscle relaxation can further enhance your stress-relief efforts. These practices encourage physical relaxation and mental clarity, helping you develop a sense of calm and balance.

Developing Resilience and Adaptability

Resilience is the ability to bounce back from challenges, setbacks, and adversity. Developing resilience is essential for navigating the ups and downs of college life. As you encounter stressors, cultivating a resilient mindset will empower you to view challenges as opportunities for growth rather than insurmountable obstacles.

One way to build resilience is by fostering a positive outlook. Adopting a growth mindset—believing that abilities and intelligence can be developed through effort and learning—can significantly impact your approach to challenges. When faced with difficulties, remind yourself that setbacks are a natural part of the learning process. Embrace failures as valuable lessons that can lead to personal growth and development.

Another key aspect of resilience is adaptability. College life is often unpredictable, requiring students to adjust to new circumstances, schedules, and environments. Embracing change and being open to new experiences can help you navigate the challenges that arise. Cultivating flexibility in your mindset allows you to adapt your plans and strategies as needed, fostering a sense of empowerment and control.

Additionally, self-compassion plays a vital role in resilience. Practicing self-compassion involves treating yourself with kindness and understanding during challenging times. Instead of being overly critical or harsh with yourself, acknowledge that everyone faces difficulties and struggles. By offering yourself compassion, you can create a supportive internal dialogue that fosters resilience.

Building a resilient support system is equally important. Surrounding yourself with individuals who uplift and encourage you can provide the strength needed to navigate challenges. Seek out friends, mentors, or counselors who understand your experiences and can offer guidance and support. Connecting with others who share similar struggles can foster a sense of community and reduce feelings of isolation.

Strategies for Healthy Time Management

Effective time management is crucial for reducing stress and achieving a balanced college experience. Learning how to allocate your time wisely can alleviate the pressure of looming deadlines and create space for self-care and relaxation. Begin by identifying your priorities and establishing a realistic schedule that reflects your commitments.

Consider using a planner or digital calendar to map out your academic responsibilities, social events, and personal time. Break larger projects into smaller, manageable tasks, and allocate specific time slots for each. This structured approach not only enhances productivity but also prevents last-minute cramming and the stress associated with procrastination.

Recognize the importance of setting boundaries. While socializing and participating in extracurricular activities are vital aspects of college life, it's essential to ensure that these commitments do not overwhelm your academic responsibilities. Learn to say no when necessary, prioritizing your health and well-being above social obligations.

Incorporating breaks into your schedule is another effective strategy for managing time and reducing stress. Allowing yourself short breaks during study sessions can enhance focus and prevent burnout. Use these breaks to engage in activities that bring you joy or relaxation, whether that's going for a walk, listening to music, or practicing mindfulness.

Finally, evaluate your progress regularly. At the end of each week, take time to reflect on what worked well and what could be improved in your time management strategies. This self-assessment will help you identify patterns and make necessary adjustments, ultimately enhancing your ability to manage your time effectively.

The Importance of Social Support and Community

Building a strong support network is vital for navigating the challenges of college life. Social support plays a significant role in reducing stress and enhancing overall well-being. Connecting with others who share similar experiences can foster a sense of belonging and provide encouragement during difficult times.

Engaging in campus activities, clubs, or organizations can be an excellent way to meet new people and establish connections. Finding communities that resonate with your interests can provide a sense of purpose and fulfillment, enhancing your college experience. These social interactions can serve as a buffer against stress, offering emotional support and camaraderie.

Additionally, don't hesitate to reach out for help when needed. Seeking support from friends, family, or campus resources is a sign of strength, not weakness. College can be overwhelming, and asking for help is a crucial step in maintaining your mental health. Whether it's talking to a trusted friend or seeking guidance from a counselor, accessing support can make a significant difference in your overall well-being.

Chapter 3: Nutrition for Mind and Body

Nutrition plays a fundamental role in supporting both physical health and mental clarity, especially during the demanding years of college. With busy schedules and limited resources, it can be challenging for students to prioritize healthy eating. However, understanding the basics of nutrition and its impact on your overall well-being is essential for thriving during this pivotal time. This chapter will explore the fundamentals of nutrition, practical tips for healthy eating on a budget, and strategies for mindful eating that can enhance your college experience.

As you navigate the pressures of academics, social life, and personal responsibilities, maintaining a balanced diet becomes increasingly important. Proper nutrition not only fuels your body but also influences your mood, energy levels, and cognitive function. By adopting healthy eating habits, you can enhance your mental clarity, improve your focus, and promote overall well-being.

Basics of Nutrition and Its Impact on Mental Clarity

Understanding the basics of nutrition is crucial for making informed food choices. Nutrients are essential for the body's functioning and can be categorized into macronutrients and micronutrients. Macronutrients include carbohydrates, proteins, and fats, which provide energy and are necessary for growth and repair. Micronutrients, including vitamins and minerals, play vital roles in various bodily functions, including brain health.

A balanced diet that includes a variety of nutrient-dense foods is key to optimizing mental clarity. Carbohydrates are particularly important, as they are the brain's primary energy source. Choosing whole grains, fruits, and vegetables can provide the necessary fuel for cognitive function while avoiding the crashes associated with processed sugars.

Proteins are essential for neurotransmitter production, which affects mood and mental clarity. Incorporating sources of lean protein, such as beans, lentils, tofu, chicken, and fish, can help support optimal brain function. Fats, particularly omega-3 fatty acids found in fatty fish, flaxseeds, and walnuts, have been linked to improved cognitive performance and emotional health.

Furthermore, hydration plays a crucial role in maintaining mental clarity. Dehydration can lead to fatigue, decreased focus, and impaired cognitive function. Aim to drink plenty of water throughout the day, especially if you're engaging in physical activities or spending long hours studying.

Healthy Eating on a College Budget

Eating healthy on a college budget is entirely possible with some planning and creativity. Many students face financial constraints that can make it challenging to prioritize nutritious foods. However, with the right strategies, you can enjoy a balanced diet without breaking the bank.

One effective approach is to create a grocery list before shopping. Planning meals for the week can help you identify what you need and reduce impulse purchases. Stick to whole foods such as fruits, vegetables, grains, and proteins, which are often more cost-effective than processed or pre-packaged items. Shopping in bulk for staples like rice, beans, and oats can also save money over time.

Consider buying seasonal produce, as it tends to be more affordable and fresher. Farmers' markets and local grocery stores often offer discounts on seasonal fruits and vegetables, making it easier to incorporate a variety of colors into your meals. Frozen fruits and vegetables are also a great option, as they retain their nutritional value and can be more budget-friendly than fresh produce.

Meal prepping is another effective strategy for healthy eating on a budget. Preparing meals in advance can save time and money while ensuring you have nutritious options readily available. Spend a few hours each week cooking and portioning out meals for the upcoming days. This practice can help prevent the temptation to resort to unhealthy takeout options during busy weeks.

In addition, consider exploring campus resources such as food pantries or community programs that offer assistance. Many colleges have initiatives to support students facing food insecurity, ensuring you have access to nutritious options.

Planning Quick, Balanced Meals and Snacks

Balancing your meals doesn't have to be complicated or time-consuming. Simple, quick meals can be nutritious and satisfying, providing you with the energy needed for your busy college lifestyle. The key is to focus on variety and balance in your meals.

A well-balanced plate typically includes a source of protein, healthy fats, carbohydrates, and plenty of colorful fruits and vegetables. For example, a quick meal could consist of a whole-grain wrap filled with grilled chicken or chickpeas, mixed greens, avocado, and a spread of hummus. This combination provides a mix of nutrients that can sustain your energy levels throughout the day.

Snacking can also play a significant role in maintaining energy and preventing hunger between meals. Opt for wholesome snacks such as Greek yogurt with fruit, nuts and seeds, or cut-up veggies with hummus. These options provide a good balance of protein, fiber, and healthy fats to keep you satisfied and focused.

Consider incorporating breakfast into your daily routine, as it can set the tone for your day. Overnight oats, smoothies, or scrambled eggs with veggies can be prepared quickly and offer a nutritious start. Aim for options that include complex carbohydrates, protein, and healthy fats to sustain your energy levels.

Batch cooking can be an efficient way to ensure you have balanced meals throughout the week. Preparing large quantities of soups, stews, or grain bowls can save time and reduce the likelihood of reaching for unhealthy convenience foods. Store leftovers in portioned containers for easy access during busy days.

Reducing Sugar and Caffeine While Staying Energized

Many college students rely on sugar and caffeine for quick energy boosts, but excessive consumption can lead to crashes and affect overall health. Learning to reduce these substances while still maintaining energy levels is essential for achieving optimal wellness.

Instead of reaching for sugary snacks or energy drinks, consider healthier alternatives. Natural sources of energy, such as fruits, nuts, and whole grains, can provide sustained energy without the crash associated with refined sugars. When you feel the urge for a sweet treat, opt for fresh fruit, which contains natural sugars along with fiber, vitamins, and minerals.

If you rely on caffeine to stay awake, consider limiting your intake and finding alternatives. While a moderate amount of caffeine can enhance focus, excessive consumption can lead to increased anxiety and disrupt sleep patterns. Instead of coffee or energy drinks, try herbal teas or infused water with citrus and mint for a refreshing boost.

Incorporating regular physical activity into your routine can also help regulate energy levels. Exercise stimulates the release of endorphins, providing a natural energy boost while reducing feelings of fatigue. Aim for short bursts of activity throughout your day, such as taking a walk between classes or participating in a quick workout session.

Sleep is another critical factor in maintaining energy levels. Prioritizing restful sleep helps your body recover and recharge, enhancing cognitive function and overall well-being. Aim for 7-9 hours of quality sleep each night and establish a calming bedtime routine to support healthy sleep habits.

Tips for Mindful Eating and Meal Prepping

Practicing mindful eating can significantly improve your relationship with food and enhance your overall well-being. Mindful eating involves being fully present during meals, paying attention to hunger cues, and savoring each bite. This approach encourages a deeper connection with food and helps prevent overeating or emotional eating.

Start by creating a calming environment for your meals. Set aside distractions, such as your phone or television, and focus solely on your food. Take the time to appreciate the colors, textures, and flavors of your meal. Chew slowly and savor each bite, allowing your body to recognize when it feels satisfied.

Incorporating meal prepping into your routine can also support mindful eating. By preparing meals in advance, you can make healthier choices and avoid impulsive eating. Consider dedicating a specific time each week for meal prep, where you can wash and chop vegetables, cook grains, and portion out meals for the week ahead.

Experiment with different recipes and cooking methods to keep your meals exciting. Variety is essential for maintaining a balanced diet and preventing boredom. Explore new ingredients, flavors, and cuisines that resonate with your taste preferences.

Lastly, be kind to yourself in your eating journey. If you have a day where you indulge in less healthy choices, recognize it as a part of life rather than a setback. Practice self-compassion and focus on getting back to balanced eating the following day.

As you continue to explore nutrition and its impact on your mind and body, remember that small changes can lead to significant improvements. By adopting healthy eating habits, you can enhance your college experience and cultivate a lifestyle that supports your holistic health.

Chapter 4: Optimizing Sleep and Rest

Sleep is one of the most critical aspects of maintaining overall health, particularly for college students who often juggle demanding schedules, academic pressures, and social commitments. Unfortunately, sleep often takes a backseat to the numerous responsibilities that come with college life, leading to fatigue, decreased cognitive performance, and increased stress levels. This chapter will explore the importance of sleep for memory and performance, provide practical tips for creating a sleep-friendly environment, and offer strategies for improving sleep quality even amid a busy lifestyle.

Understanding the role of sleep in your daily functioning is essential for optimizing your health. Quality rest not only enhances memory consolidation but also impacts mood, energy levels, and overall well-being. By prioritizing sleep and implementing effective strategies to improve your sleep habits, you can significantly enhance your academic performance and daily life.

Why Sleep Is Essential for Memory and Performance

Research consistently demonstrates that sleep plays a vital role in cognitive function, including memory, learning, and problem-solving. During sleep, particularly during the rapid eye movement (REM) phase, the brain processes and consolidates information gathered throughout the day. This process is essential for transforming short-term memories into long-term ones, allowing you to retain knowledge and perform better academically.

Sleep deprivation can lead to impaired cognitive function, including difficulty concentrating, reduced attention span, and slower reaction times. For college students, this can have serious implications, particularly during exams or important assignments. A lack of adequate rest can also impact your mood, increasing the likelihood of stress and anxiety, which further hinders academic performance.

Moreover, sleep affects physical health, including immune function, hormonal balance, and metabolic regulation. Inadequate sleep can contribute to various health issues, including obesity, diabetes, and cardiovascular problems. For students aiming for optimal performance, prioritizing sleep is crucial for maintaining both mental and physical health.

Creating a Sleep-Friendly Environment in Dorms

The environment in which you sleep can significantly impact the quality of your rest. Creating a sleep-friendly environment in your dorm can help foster better sleep habits and improve overall sleep quality. Here are some essential tips for transforming your dorm room into a restful haven.

First, consider the lighting in your space. Exposure to bright lights, particularly blue light from screens, can interfere with your body's natural circadian rhythm. Aim to limit screen time at least an hour before bedtime. Use blackout curtains or eye masks to minimize outside light and create a dark environment conducive to sleep. If you must use artificial light, opt for soft, warm lighting in the evening.

Noise can also disrupt your sleep. If your dorm is in a busy area or near common spaces, consider using earplugs or a white noise machine to drown out distracting sounds. Soft background noise can help create a calming atmosphere that promotes relaxation.

Temperature is another crucial factor in creating a sleep-friendly environment. The ideal sleep temperature varies from person to person, but most people find that a cooler room (around 60-67°F or 15-19°C) promotes better sleep.

Adjust your thermostat or use a fan to maintain a comfortable temperature throughout the night.

Additionally, invest in comfortable bedding. A supportive mattress and pillows that suit your sleeping position can make a significant difference in sleep quality. Choose soft, breathable sheets and blankets to enhance comfort. Create a cozy sleep space that encourages relaxation and rest.

Tips for Better Sleep, Even with a Busy Schedule

Balancing a hectic college schedule can make it challenging to prioritize sleep, but there are practical strategies you can implement to improve your sleep quality despite a busy lifestyle. One key approach is to establish a consistent sleep routine. Going to bed and waking up at the same time each day, even on weekends, helps regulate your body's internal clock and promotes better sleep.

Consider creating a calming pre-sleep ritual that signals to your body that it's time to wind down. This can include activities such as reading, gentle stretching, or practicing relaxation techniques like meditation or deep breathing. Engaging in these calming activities before bed can help reduce stress and prepare your mind and body for sleep.

If you find yourself needing to study late into the night, try to incorporate short breaks to maintain focus and energy.

The Pomodoro technique—working for 25 minutes, followed by a 5-minute break—can help you stay productive without sacrificing sleep. During breaks, engage in light stretching or deep breathing exercises to refresh your mind and body.

Avoid consuming caffeine and heavy meals close to bedtime, as both can interfere with your ability to fall asleep. Instead, opt for light snacks if you feel hungry in the evening. Foods rich in magnesium, such as bananas or nuts, can promote relaxation and aid sleep.

Lastly, if you find yourself overwhelmed with assignments or exams, don't hesitate to reach out for support. Many colleges offer resources such as counseling services, academic advisors, and workshops that can help you manage your stress and develop effective time management skills.

Power Naps: How to Use Them Effectively

When faced with the challenges of a busy schedule, power naps can be a valuable tool for enhancing alertness and cognitive performance. A short nap of 20 to 30 minutes can help refresh your mind without causing grogginess or interfering with your nighttime sleep.

To make the most of power naps, choose a comfortable spot where you can relax without distractions. Use an alarm to ensure you don't oversleep, and keep your naps early in the day to avoid disrupting your nighttime sleep schedule. Napping too late in the afternoon can leave you feeling energized when it's time to wind down for the night.

If you find it difficult to fall asleep during the day, consider incorporating relaxation techniques such as deep breathing or visualization before napping. This can help calm your mind and prepare your body for a restful short sleep.

While power naps can provide temporary relief, they should not replace adequate nighttime sleep. Use them as a supplementary tool to manage fatigue, especially during particularly demanding weeks or after late-night study sessions.

Recognizing and Addressing Sleep Disorders

While many college students experience temporary sleep disturbances, persistent sleep issues may indicate an underlying sleep disorder. Common disorders such as insomnia, sleep apnea, and restless leg syndrome can significantly impact your overall health and well-being.

Recognizing the signs of a sleep disorder is crucial for addressing the issue effectively. If you frequently have difficulty falling asleep, staying asleep, or feel excessively tired during the day despite adequate sleep, consider consulting a healthcare professional. They can help assess your symptoms, provide appropriate guidance, and recommend potential treatments.

Implementing healthy sleep habits is often an effective first step in addressing sleep disorders. However, in some cases, more specialized interventions may be necessary. Treatment options may include cognitive-behavioral therapy (CBT), medication, or lifestyle changes tailored to your specific needs.

If you suspect you have sleep apnea, which is characterized by interruptions in breathing during sleep, seek medical evaluation promptly. This condition can have serious implications for your overall health if left untreated.

Ultimately, prioritizing sleep and recognizing the importance of rest is vital for academic success and overall well-being. By adopting healthy sleep habits, creating a supportive sleep environment, and addressing any persistent sleep issues, you can enhance your college experience and foster a balanced, healthy lifestyle.

Chapter 5: Physical Activity and Movement

Physical activity plays a crucial role in maintaining overall health and well-being, especially for college students navigating the demands of academics, social life, and personal responsibilities. Regular exercise not only supports physical health but also enhances mental clarity, boosts mood, and helps to manage stress. This chapter will explore the myriad benefits of incorporating physical activity into your daily routine, provide practical types of exercises that fit into a busy college lifestyle, and share strategies for staying motivated to stay active.

Understanding the importance of movement is essential for fostering a balanced and healthy life during your college years. While it can be tempting to prioritize studying or socializing over physical activity, recognizing that exercise contributes significantly to your academic success and emotional well-being is key. By integrating regular movement into your routine, you can create a foundation for long-term health that will benefit you both during and after your college experience.

Benefits of Regular Exercise for Mood and Focus

Engaging in regular physical activity offers numerous benefits for both mental and emotional health. Exercise is known to stimulate the production of endorphins, often referred to as "feel-good" hormones. These chemicals interact with receptors in your brain to reduce the perception of pain and trigger a positive feeling in the body, promoting an improved mood. This effect can be especially valuable for college students, who may experience periods of stress, anxiety, or depressive symptoms due to academic pressures and life transitions.

Additionally, exercise can enhance cognitive function, leading to improved focus and concentration. Studies have shown that regular physical activity increases blood flow to the brain, promoting better oxygen and nutrient delivery. This, in turn, can help enhance memory, creativity, and overall cognitive performance. For students facing long study sessions or preparing for exams, incorporating movement into your day can provide the mental boost you need to stay sharp and alert.

Furthermore, exercise can help regulate sleep patterns, which is particularly important for college students often juggling erratic schedules. Improved sleep quality enhances your ability to concentrate during the day and contributes to better academic performance. By fostering a consistent exercise routine, you create a positive feedback loop that supports both physical and mental well-being.

Types of Exercises That Fit Into a College Routine

Incorporating physical activity into a busy college routine doesn't have to be complicated or time-consuming. There are various types of exercises that can easily fit into your day, regardless of your schedule or fitness level. Finding activities you enjoy will make it easier to stay committed to regular movement.

Cardiovascular exercises, such as jogging, cycling, or brisk walking, are excellent ways to increase heart rate and improve endurance. Many college campuses offer opportunities for group workouts or access to recreational facilities where students can engage in cardio activities. Even short bouts of cardio—like a 15-minute walk between classes—can be effective in boosting energy levels and improving mood.

Strength training is another crucial component of a balanced fitness routine. Bodyweight exercises, such as push-ups, squats, and lunges, can be performed anywhere and require no equipment, making them ideal for college students. Resistance bands are also a portable and cost-effective option for strength training, allowing you to challenge your muscles with various exercises that can be completed in a small space.

Flexibility and balance exercises, like yoga or Pilates, can help improve your posture, reduce tension, and enhance overall well-being. Many universities offer fitness classes that incorporate these modalities, making it easy to explore new activities and find what works for you. Alternatively, numerous online platforms provide guided sessions that you can do in your dorm room.

For students who enjoy socializing, team sports can be an excellent way to stay active while connecting with peers. Intramural sports leagues and recreational teams are often available on college campuses, providing a fun and engaging environment for exercise. These activities not only promote physical fitness but also foster community and camaraderie among participants.

Simple Workouts You Can Do in Small Spaces

Living in a dorm or a small apartment doesn't mean you can't maintain an effective workout routine. Many simple workouts can be performed in limited space, allowing you to stay active without needing a gym or large exercise area. The key is to focus on bodyweight exercises that utilize your own weight for resistance.

High-intensity interval training (HIIT) is a popular workout style that involves short bursts of intense exercise followed by brief rest periods. HIIT workouts can be tailored to fit any space and require minimal equipment. For example, you might incorporate exercises like jumping jacks, burpees, mountain climbers, and planks into a 20-minute HIIT routine that you can do right in your room.

If you prefer a more structured approach, consider creating a circuit workout. Select five to six bodyweight exercises and perform them consecutively with little rest in between. For instance, you could create a circuit that includes squats, push-ups, tricep dips, high knees, and lunges. Repeat the circuit two to three times for a full-body workout.

For stretching and flexibility, dedicated yoga or Pilates sessions can be easily conducted in a small space. Many online resources provide guided workouts, allowing you to follow along from the comfort of your dorm. These practices not only improve flexibility and balance but also provide an opportunity to relax and reduce stress.

Balancing Exercise with Academics and Social Life

Finding time to exercise amid the demands of academic coursework and social activities can be challenging, but striking a balance is essential for overall well-being. Start by assessing your weekly schedule and identifying pockets of time that can be dedicated to physical activity. Whether it's a morning run, a workout during breaks, or an evening yoga session, prioritizing movement can enhance your productivity and mood.

One effective strategy for maintaining balance is to combine social interactions with physical activity. Invite friends to join you for a workout, a hike, or a group sports game. This not only helps you stay active but also strengthens your social connections. Creating a fitness group or joining workout classes together can foster accountability and motivation.

It's also essential to listen to your body and recognize when you need to prioritize rest over exercise. While staying active is crucial, ensuring you don't overexert yourself is equally important. Pay attention to signs of fatigue or burnout, and allow yourself to take breaks or modify your workouts as needed. Ultimately, maintaining a flexible approach to fitness will help you integrate physical activity into your life sustainably.

How to Stay Motivated to Stay Active

Staying motivated to maintain an active lifestyle can be challenging, especially during busy or stressful times. However, there are several strategies you can use to cultivate motivation and make exercise a regular part of your routine. First, set realistic and achievable goals that align with your interests and lifestyle. Rather than aiming for perfection, focus on small, incremental changes that you can build upon over time.

Keeping track of your progress can also enhance motivation. Use a fitness app, journal, or calendar to log your workouts and achievements. Celebrating milestones, no matter how small, can boost your confidence and inspire you to continue. Additionally, consider finding a workout buddy or accountability partner who shares your fitness goals. Exercising together can provide support, encouragement, and a sense of camaraderie.

Incorporate variety into your workouts to keep things fresh and exciting. Experiment with new classes, outdoor activities, or sports that pique your interest. This not only helps prevent boredom but also allows you to discover new passions that can enhance your fitness journey.

Lastly, remind yourself of the benefits of physical activity and how it positively impacts your life. Reflect on how exercise improves your mood, reduces stress, and enhances your overall well-being. By focusing on the positive outcomes of staying active, you can maintain motivation and commitment to your health and wellness goals.

Chapter 6: Mental Health and Emotional Well-being

College life is an exciting yet challenging experience that can take a significant toll on mental health. Many students face unique stressors that can lead to mental health challenges, including anxiety, depression, and feelings of isolation. Recognizing these challenges is the first step toward fostering emotional well-being during this pivotal period. This chapter delves into the common mental health issues students encounter, practical techniques for managing these challenges, the significance of self-compassion and positive self-talk, and the resources available on campus for mental health support. Additionally, we will explore how mindfulness practices can help build emotional resilience.

Understanding mental health is essential for maintaining a balanced life while navigating the demands of college. Many students may feel overwhelmed by coursework, social pressures, or the transition to independence, and it's vital to acknowledge that these feelings are common and valid. By equipping yourself with the right tools and knowledge, you can cultivate a positive mindset and navigate the complexities of college life with greater ease.

Understanding Common Mental Health Challenges in College

Mental health challenges among college students are widespread, with many experiencing anxiety and depression at some point during their academic journey. According to various studies, a significant percentage of students report feeling overwhelmed by their responsibilities, leading to symptoms of anxiety and depression. The pressures of academic performance, social dynamics, and financial concerns can contribute to these feelings, making it crucial for students to be aware of their mental health and seek help when needed.

Anxiety is often characterized by excessive worry or fear, and college students may experience it in various forms—social anxiety, test anxiety, or general anxiety related to the uncertainties of adulthood. The fear of failure or not meeting expectations can exacerbate these feelings, leading to a cycle of stress that can impact academic performance and overall well-being. It's essential to recognize the signs of anxiety and understand that seeking support is a strength, not a weakness.

Depression, on the other hand, may manifest as persistent sadness, a lack of interest in activities, or difficulty concentrating. Many students may dismiss these feelings as typical stress or fatigue, but it's vital to differentiate between temporary emotional fluctuations and more serious mental health issues. Understanding the symptoms of depression and acknowledging their impact on daily life can help students take proactive steps toward recovery and self-care.

Techniques for Managing Anxiety and Depression

Managing anxiety and depression requires a multifaceted approach, as no single technique will work for everyone. However, there are several practical strategies that can help alleviate symptoms and promote emotional well-being. One effective method is establishing a routine. Routines provide structure and predictability, which can be especially beneficial for students facing an overwhelming array of responsibilities. Setting specific times for studying, socializing, and self-care can create a sense of control and stability.

Physical activity also plays a significant role in managing anxiety and depression. As discussed in the previous chapter, regular exercise releases endorphins that improve mood and reduce feelings of stress. Finding enjoyable physical activities—whether it's joining a campus sports team, participating in group workouts, or taking a daily walk—can have profound effects on mental health.

Mindfulness practices are another powerful tool for managing anxiety and depression. Techniques such as meditation, deep breathing exercises, and yoga can help ground students in the present moment, reducing the tendency to ruminate on negative thoughts or future uncertainties. Setting aside even a few minutes each day for mindfulness can lead to greater emotional clarity and resilience.

Additionally, journaling can be a valuable practice for processing emotions and reducing anxiety. Writing about your feelings, experiences, and thoughts can provide an outlet for self-expression and help you gain perspective on your challenges. Reflecting on positive experiences or expressing gratitude in your journal can also shift your focus from negativity to appreciation.

The Importance of Self-Compassion and Positive Self-Talk

In the face of academic pressures and personal challenges, practicing self-compassion is essential. Many students are their harshest critics, often holding themselves to unrealistic standards. Learning to treat yourself with kindness and understanding can significantly impact your mental health. Instead of berating yourself for perceived shortcomings, try to approach your struggles with empathy. Recognize that everyone experiences difficulties, and it's okay to make mistakes.

Positive self-talk is another critical component of mental well-being. The way you talk to yourself influences your mood and self-esteem. Replacing negative thoughts with positive affirmations can help create a more supportive inner dialogue. For instance, instead of thinking, "I can't do this," try reframing it to "I am doing my best, and I will figure this out." This shift in mindset can empower you to approach challenges with greater confidence and resilience.

Cultivating self-compassion and positive self-talk requires practice, but the rewards are immense. As you learn to treat yourself with kindness and support, you'll find it easier to navigate the ups and downs of college life without becoming overwhelmed.

Resources on Campus for Mental Health Support

Most colleges and universities offer a variety of resources to support students' mental health. These resources may include counseling services, workshops, support groups, and mental health awareness campaigns. If you're struggling with mental health challenges, reaching out for support is crucial. Many campuses have trained professionals who can provide guidance, counseling, and coping strategies tailored to your individual needs.

Counseling centers often offer one-on-one sessions with licensed counselors, providing a safe and confidential space to discuss your thoughts and feelings. These professionals can help you develop coping mechanisms, explore underlying issues, and create a personalized plan for mental wellness. Additionally, many campuses offer group therapy or support groups, where students can connect with others facing similar challenges.

It's essential to take advantage of these resources and not hesitate to seek help. College can be a stressful and transformative time, and you don't have to navigate it alone. Many students find that discussing their struggles with a professional can provide clarity and relief, allowing them to approach their studies and personal life with renewed focus.

Building Emotional Resilience Through Mindfulness Practices

Mindfulness is a practice that encourages individuals to stay present and engaged in the moment, cultivating awareness and acceptance of their thoughts and feelings. Building emotional resilience through mindfulness practices can help students better manage stress and bounce back from setbacks. Incorporating mindfulness into your daily routine can be as simple as taking a few moments to focus on your breath, practicing guided meditation, or engaging in mindful movement like yoga.

Mindfulness exercises encourage you to observe your thoughts without judgment, allowing you to gain insight into your emotional responses. This practice can help break the cycle of negative thinking that often accompanies anxiety and depression. Over time, mindfulness fosters greater emotional resilience, enabling you to respond to challenges with a sense of calm and clarity.

Moreover, mindfulness encourages self-acceptance and appreciation for the present moment. By learning to embrace your current experience, you can cultivate gratitude and positivity, even in the face of adversity. Many students find that mindfulness practices not only enhance their mental well-being but also improve their overall quality of life during college.

Mental health and emotional well-being are critical components of a holistic approach to health in college. By understanding the common challenges students face, employing practical techniques for managing anxiety and depression, practicing self-compassion, utilizing campus resources, and embracing mindfulness, you can cultivate a positive and resilient mindset. These skills will not only help you navigate your college years but will also serve as valuable tools for lifelong wellness.

Chapter 7: Social Connections and Building a Supportive Community

Social health plays a pivotal role in our overall well-being, particularly during the transformative years of college. For many students, college represents not only an academic journey but also a unique opportunity to forge lasting relationships and connections. However, the transition to this new environment can be challenging, leading to feelings of isolation, homesickness, and stress. In this chapter, we will explore the importance of social health and connection, strategies for finding your community on campus, navigating social pressures, building and maintaining healthy relationships, and coping with homesickness and loneliness.

As social beings, humans thrive on connections with others. These connections can provide emotional support, foster a sense of belonging, and enhance overall happiness. College is a time to explore diverse social circles and develop meaningful relationships, but it's essential to approach this journey with intention and awareness. By actively cultivating a supportive community, you can navigate the challenges of college life more effectively and enrich your overall experience.

The Importance of Social Health and Connection

Social health encompasses our ability to form meaningful relationships and connect with others in a way that enhances our emotional and mental well-being. Strong social ties can lead to improved mood, reduced stress, and better overall health. Research indicates that individuals with robust social networks experience lower levels of anxiety and depression, greater resilience in the face of challenges, and even improved physical health.

In college, the importance of social connections becomes even more pronounced. The transition to campus life can be overwhelming, as students may leave behind familiar support systems. Establishing new relationships and finding a sense of community can mitigate feelings of loneliness and help students adapt to their new environment. Social connections can provide a buffer against the pressures of academic life and create a supportive atmosphere for personal growth.

Moreover, engaging with peers can foster a sense of belonging, which is vital for emotional well-being. When students feel connected to their peers and campus community, they are more likely to thrive academically and personally. Positive social interactions can enhance motivation, boost self-esteem, and create a network of support that promotes resilience in the face of challenges.

Finding Your Community on Campus

Finding your community on campus requires intentional effort and exploration. Many colleges and universities offer a wide range of clubs, organizations, and activities designed to help students connect with like-minded individuals. Whether you're interested in joining a sports team, participating in cultural clubs, or engaging in community service, there are numerous opportunities to meet new people who share your interests.

Start by exploring the campus activities fair or joining student organizations that resonate with your passions. These gatherings provide a great chance to meet fellow students and discover shared interests. If you're unsure where to start, consider reflecting on your hobbies or activities that excite you. Engaging in activities you genuinely enjoy can lead you to individuals with similar interests, creating a solid foundation for meaningful connections.

In addition to clubs and organizations, consider attending campus events, workshops, and social gatherings. These events are often designed to promote interaction among students and provide opportunities for networking. Don't hesitate to step out of your comfort zone and engage with new people. Building connections often requires initiative and openness, so be willing to strike up conversations and explore new friendships.

For those who may find large social settings intimidating, consider seeking smaller, more intimate gatherings. Participating in study groups, attending coffee meetups, or joining discussions in residence halls can provide a more relaxed environment for connecting with peers. Remember that building a community takes time, and it's essential to be patient as you navigate the process.

Navigating Social Pressure and Setting Boundaries

While building connections is vital, it's equally important to navigate social pressures and set boundaries that align with your values and well-being. College life can present various social dynamics, including peer pressure to engage in certain behaviors or activities. Recognizing and addressing these pressures is crucial for maintaining your mental and emotional health.

One effective strategy for navigating social pressure is to establish clear personal boundaries. Boundaries are essential for protecting your well-being and ensuring that you engage in activities that resonate with your values. Take time to reflect on what feels comfortable for you and communicate these boundaries with others. Whether it's regarding time commitments, social activities, or academic responsibilities, being clear about your limits can help you navigate social situations with confidence.

Additionally, surround yourself with individuals who respect your boundaries and support your well-being. Seek friendships with those who encourage healthy choices and contribute positively to your life. It's important to cultivate relationships that foster mutual respect, understanding, and support. If you find yourself in social situations that make you uncomfortable, don't hesitate to excuse yourself or seek alternative activities that align with your values.

Remember that it's okay to say no. Prioritizing your mental and emotional health may require declining invitations or stepping back from certain social engagements. By honoring your needs and boundaries, you'll create space for authentic connections that contribute positively to your college experience.

Building and Maintaining Healthy Relationships

Building healthy relationships involves ongoing effort and communication. As you navigate social dynamics, prioritize relationships that promote positivity, trust, and support. Healthy relationships should be reciprocal, with both individuals contributing to each other's well-being.

Effective communication is a cornerstone of healthy relationships. Be open and honest with your friends about your thoughts, feelings, and needs. Encourage your friends to share their experiences as well, fostering a safe environment for mutual understanding. Active listening is also crucial; when friends feel heard and validated, it strengthens the bond between individuals.

Additionally, make time for your friendships. Life in college can be busy, but prioritizing social connections is essential for maintaining healthy relationships. Schedule regular catch-ups with friends, whether in person or virtually, to stay connected and support each other through challenges. These moments of connection can provide a much-needed break from academic stress and reinforce your sense of community.

It's also important to recognize that relationships may evolve over time. Some friendships may grow stronger, while others may fade. Embrace these changes and be open to new connections. Building a diverse social network can enrich your college experience and expose you to various perspectives and experiences.

Coping with Homesickness and Loneliness

Feeling homesick or lonely is a common experience for many college students, especially during the initial transition to campus life. These feelings can arise from missing familiar environments, friends, and family. Acknowledging and addressing homesickness is crucial for maintaining emotional well-being.

To cope with homesickness, consider creating routines that honor your connection to home. Engaging in familiar activities, such as cooking family recipes, listening to music that reminds you of home, or maintaining contact with loved ones through video calls, can provide comfort and help ease feelings of longing.

Building a supportive community on campus can also alleviate feelings of loneliness. By actively engaging with peers and seeking new friendships, you can create a sense of belonging that mitigates homesickness. Remember that many students share similar experiences, and forming connections can provide mutual support during this transitional period.

If feelings of loneliness persist, consider reaching out to campus resources such as counseling services or support groups. These resources can offer guidance and connection, helping you navigate feelings of isolation.

Don't hesitate to seek help if you find that homesickness or loneliness significantly impacts your well-being.

Social connections and building a supportive community are vital components of holistic health during college. By recognizing the importance of social health, actively seeking connections, navigating social pressures, and maintaining healthy relationships, you can cultivate a fulfilling and balanced college experience. Embracing the challenges of social dynamics and prioritizing emotional well-being will ultimately contribute to your overall success and happiness as you navigate this transformative time in your life.

Chapter 8: Academic Balance and Study Strategies

Navigating the academic landscape of college can be both exhilarating and overwhelming. With rigorous coursework, looming deadlines, and high expectations, it's easy for students to find themselves in a cycle of stress and anxiety. Academic pressure can significantly impact overall health, leading to feelings of burnout, fatigue, and even mental health challenges. This chapter will explore how academic stress affects well-being, effective study habits and focus techniques, the importance of balancing academics with self-care, strategies to prevent burnout, and the value of utilizing academic resources and support systems.

In a college setting, students often feel compelled to excel academically, which can create an immense burden. However, understanding how to manage academic demands without sacrificing personal health is crucial for long-term success. By adopting effective study strategies and maintaining a healthy balance, students can foster a more enjoyable and fulfilling academic experience.

How Academic Stress Impacts Overall Health

Academic stress is a pervasive issue among college students. The pressure to achieve high grades, complete assignments on time, and prepare for exams can lead to heightened anxiety levels. Prolonged stress can manifest physically and mentally, causing headaches, fatigue, digestive issues, and sleep disturbances. Moreover, chronic academic stress can contribute to feelings of inadequacy and self-doubt, undermining overall self-esteem.

Understanding the relationship between academic stress and health is essential. When stress levels rise, the body's fight-or-flight response is triggered, releasing hormones like cortisol and adrenaline. While this response can be beneficial in short bursts, chronic activation can lead to negative health outcomes. For students, this can mean decreased focus, impaired memory, and a reduced ability to retain information.

Furthermore, the competitive nature of college can create an environment where stress is normalized. Many students may feel pressured to sacrifice their well-being in pursuit of academic success, often neglecting self-care practices. It is crucial to recognize that academic excellence should not come at the cost of physical and mental health. By addressing academic stress proactively, students can create a healthier balance that supports both their educational and personal goals.

Effective Study Habits and Focus Techniques

Developing effective study habits is key to managing academic stress and enhancing performance. Students should start by creating a dedicated study environment that minimizes distractions and promotes concentration. A clutter-free space, adequate lighting, and comfortable seating can make a significant difference in focus and productivity. Personalizing the study area with motivational quotes or items that inspire creativity can also boost morale.

Time management is another critical component of effective studying. Students should create a study schedule that allocates specific times for different subjects or tasks. Breaking study sessions into manageable chunks can help prevent feelings of overwhelm. Techniques like the Pomodoro Technique, which involves studying for 25 minutes followed by a 5-minute break, can enhance focus and retention.

Additionally, students should consider varying their study methods. Active learning strategies, such as summarizing material in your own words, teaching concepts to peers, or utilizing flashcards, can enhance retention and understanding. Incorporating multimedia resources, such as videos or podcasts, can also make studying more engaging.

Another effective technique is to establish study groups. Collaborating with peers not only fosters accountability but also encourages the exchange of ideas and perspectives. Explaining concepts to others reinforces understanding and can clarify difficult topics. However, it's essential to strike a balance; while group study can be beneficial, it's crucial to ensure that the group remains focused and productive.

Maintaining Balance Between Academics and Self-Care

Maintaining a balance between academic responsibilities and self-care is vital for overall health. Students often underestimate the importance of incorporating self-care practices into their routines, leading to burnout and diminished well-being. Self-care can take many forms, including physical activity, mindfulness practices, and hobbies that bring joy.

Scheduling regular breaks during study sessions is crucial for mental clarity. Short breaks allow students to recharge and refocus, preventing mental fatigue. Incorporating physical activity into daily routines, even in small doses, can significantly improve mood and energy levels. Whether it's a quick walk around campus, a dance break in your room, or a short workout, movement helps alleviate stress and boosts productivity.

Mindfulness practices, such as meditation or deep breathing exercises, can also promote balance. Taking just a few minutes each day to practice mindfulness can help students manage stress and maintain clarity. Mindfulness enhances awareness of thoughts and feelings, allowing for better emotional regulation during challenging academic moments.

Moreover, students should not shy away from pursuing hobbies or interests outside of their academic workload. Engaging in activities that bring joy, whether it's painting, playing an instrument, or participating in a sport, fosters a sense of fulfillment that complements academic achievements. Balancing academic demands with personal interests can lead to a more well-rounded and enriching college experience.

Preventing Burnout Through Strategic Planning

Burnout is a state of emotional, physical, and mental exhaustion caused by prolonged stress. In a college setting, students may experience burnout due to overwhelming academic workloads, inadequate self-care, and unrealistic expectations. Preventing burnout requires proactive strategies and careful planning.

Students should prioritize self-awareness by regularly assessing their workload and stress levels. Recognizing signs of burnout, such as fatigue, irritability, and disengagement, is essential. When students notice these signs, it may be time to reevaluate commitments and adjust expectations.

Strategic planning plays a crucial role in preventing burnout. Creating a semester plan that outlines deadlines, exams, and personal commitments can help students anticipate busy periods and allocate time for self-care. Setting realistic goals for assignments and study sessions ensures that students do not overload themselves with tasks.

Additionally, seeking balance in course selection can alleviate academic pressure. Students should strive for a well-rounded schedule that includes a mix of challenging and manageable courses. By diversifying their workload, students can avoid overwhelming themselves with intensive courses in a single semester.

Incorporating regular check-ins with academic advisors or mentors can also provide valuable support and guidance. These individuals can offer insights into course planning, time management, and strategies for success. Building a network of support enhances resilience and fosters a sense of community, which is crucial for maintaining balance during challenging times.

Using Academic Resources and Seeking Support

Colleges and universities typically offer a wealth of academic resources designed to support student success. Taking advantage of these resources can significantly alleviate stress and enhance academic performance. Libraries, writing centers, tutoring services, and study groups provide valuable assistance in navigating academic challenges.

Students should familiarize themselves with the academic resources available on their campus. Attending orientation sessions and exploring the college website can help students identify the support systems at their disposal. For example, many institutions offer free tutoring services, writing assistance, and workshops on study skills. Utilizing these resources can enhance understanding of course material and improve overall performance.

Additionally, students should not hesitate to seek support from professors and academic advisors. Professors often appreciate students who take the initiative to ask questions and seek clarification on course material. Building a rapport with faculty can lead to valuable mentorship opportunities and guidance on academic pathways.

Furthermore, peer support can be instrumental in academic success. Forming study groups with classmates can foster collaboration and mutual motivation. Engaging in discussions with peers not only enhances understanding of complex topics but also creates a sense of camaraderie that can make studying more enjoyable.

Achieving academic balance and implementing effective study strategies are essential for holistic health in college. By understanding the impacts of academic stress on overall well-being, adopting effective study habits, prioritizing self-care, preventing burnout through strategic planning, and utilizing academic resources, students can navigate their academic journeys with greater ease.

Chapter 9: Avoiding Substance Misuse and Making Healthy Choices

Navigating the college experience often involves a complex interplay of social pressures and personal choices. As students immerse themselves in this vibrant, sometimes overwhelming environment, they frequently encounter various substances that promise to enhance their social lives or relieve stress. However, understanding the implications of substance use is crucial for maintaining your health and well-being. This chapter explores the common pressures related to substance use in college, the effects of alcohol and drugs on health, effective strategies for managing social pressure, building confidence in your choices, and finding fun and relaxation without resorting to substances.

College is often depicted as a carefree time filled with parties, late nights, and spontaneous adventures. This narrative can create a sense of obligation to partake in drinking and drug use as a rite of passage. Many students feel that they must conform to social norms and engage in substance use to fit in with their peers. This perception can lead to a cycle of pressure where the desire to belong outweighs the need for personal health and safety. Recognizing this dynamic is the first step toward empowering yourself to make informed choices.

Common Substance-Related Pressures in College

Substance-related pressures can manifest in various forms, often starting with the most socially accepted ones, like alcohol. Parties, bar nights, and social gatherings frequently emphasize drinking as a key component of the experience. This expectation can create an environment where abstaining from alcohol feels like a deviation from the norm. Furthermore, peers may actively encourage or pressure you to partake, equating substance use with fun, acceptance, and camaraderie. For many students, this pressure can lead to uncomfortable situations where the need to socialize conflicts with personal values or health considerations.

Additionally, the prevalence of illicit drug use on many college campuses further complicates the landscape. Recreational drugs may be easily accessible, with peer pressure amplifying the allure of trying them. The social stigma surrounding refusal can make it feel challenging to decline participation. Even when a student is aware of the risks associated with these substances, the desire to fit in can overshadow better judgment.

Understanding the Effects of Alcohol and Drugs on Health

Education is crucial in combating the pressures surrounding substance use. Many students underestimate the short- and long-term effects of alcohol and drugs on their bodies and minds. Alcohol, for instance, can significantly impair cognitive function, which can hinder academic performance and memory retention. In addition to affecting grades, excessive drinking can lead to poor decision-making, accidents, and injuries. It can also have more severe health implications, such as addiction or liver damage.

Drugs, both recreational and prescription, can have even more profound effects. They can alter brain chemistry, potentially leading to dependency and mental health issues. Recreational drugs can interfere with emotional regulation, heightening feelings of anxiety or depression. Understanding these consequences is vital in making informed choices about your health and well-being. The more you know about the potential impact of these substances, the better equipped you are to resist the pressures to engage in substance use.

Tips for Handling Social Pressure Around Substances

When faced with social situations that involve substance use, having strategies to manage pressure is essential. The first step is to develop a clear understanding of your values and motivations regarding substance use. Why do you choose to abstain? Is it for health reasons, personal beliefs, or a desire to maintain focus on your academic goals? Having these reasons firmly in mind will bolster your confidence when confronted with pressure.

Practicing assertiveness is a key strategy for handling social situations. Learning to say no confidently is an essential skill that takes practice. You don't have to provide elaborate excuses or justifications for your choices; a simple, straightforward refusal can be effective. For example, saying, "I'm not drinking tonight, but thanks!" conveys your decision without inviting further discussion. It's also helpful to rehearse responses in advance, so you feel prepared when the moment arises.

Another effective strategy is to seek out like-minded individuals who share your commitment to making healthy choices. Surrounding yourself with a supportive community can provide encouragement and reinforce your decisions. When your friends value health and well-being, you're less likely to feel pressured to conform to substance-related norms. Additionally, seek out alternative social activities that do not center around alcohol or drugs. Many college campuses offer clubs, recreational sports, and events focused on healthy living that can serve as great outlets for socialization without the influence of substances.

Building Confidence to Make Healthy Decisions

Building confidence in your ability to make healthy choices requires self-reflection and practice. Acknowledge the societal pressures that exist but remember that you have the power to prioritize your health and well-being. Consider the consequences of substance use on your long-term goals. Ask yourself how engaging in drinking or drug use aligns with your vision for your future. Visualizing a successful, healthy version of yourself can help strengthen your resolve when faced with temptation.

Self-compassion is another crucial aspect of building confidence. Understand that it's normal to feel conflicted in social situations, but practicing kindness toward yourself can reduce anxiety and self-doubt. Reflect on your accomplishments, and remind yourself that choosing health is a personal victory worth celebrating.

Alternatives for Fun and Relaxation Without Substances

Finding enjoyable alternatives to substances can enrich your college experience and promote well-being. There are countless activities that foster connection and relaxation without the negative effects of alcohol or drugs. Explore options such as joining clubs, attending workshops, or participating in community service projects. Engaging in activities you genuinely enjoy can help you forge deeper connections with others and create fulfilling experiences.

Physical activities are excellent substitutes for substance use as they provide natural stress relief and promote endorphin production. Whether it's joining an intramural sports team, attending fitness classes, or practicing yoga, physical activity can offer a sense of achievement and enhance your mood. Additionally, spending time in nature—hiking, biking, or simply taking walks—can provide a refreshing break from the demands of college life.

Creative outlets, such as painting, writing, or playing music, can also serve as powerful alternatives for relaxation and expression. These activities provide a sense of purpose and accomplishment, helping to alleviate stress without the need for substances. Organizing game nights with friends, cooking together, or hosting movie marathons can also be enjoyable ways to spend time together while staying substance-free.

Avoiding substance misuse during college is essential for your overall health and well-being. By understanding the common pressures surrounding substance use, recognizing the health implications of alcohol and drugs, and implementing effective strategies for managing social situations, you can create a fulfilling college experience that prioritizes your well-being.

Building confidence in your choices, surrounding yourself with supportive friends, and exploring alternative activities will empower you to thrive during your college years and beyond. Remember, making healthy decisions now sets the foundation for a balanced, vibrant life in the future.

Chapter 10: Creating a Personal Wellness Plan

In the whirlwind of college life, it's easy to lose sight of personal health and wellness amid academic pressures, social obligations, and the quest for success. However, developing a personal wellness plan is essential for navigating these challenges while maintaining a balanced, healthy lifestyle. This chapter will guide you through assessing your needs, setting specific wellness goals, tracking your progress, and adjusting your plan as life changes. We'll also explore how to integrate wellness practices into your post-college life and emphasize the importance of staying committed to a lifelong journey of health and balance.

Assessing Your Needs and Setting Specific Wellness Goals

Creating an effective wellness plan begins with a thorough assessment of your current health status and lifestyle. Take time to reflect on your physical, emotional, and social well-being. Are there specific areas where you feel you could improve? Perhaps you're struggling with stress management, finding time to exercise, or maintaining a balanced diet. Identifying these areas of need will help you tailor your wellness goals to your unique circumstances.

To get started, consider keeping a journal for a week or two, where you can document your daily habits and feelings. Note down your meals, exercise routines, sleep patterns, and moments of stress. Pay attention to how you feel physically and emotionally throughout the day. This practice can provide you with valuable insights into your current lifestyle, helping you identify patterns or habits that may need adjusting.

Once you've assessed your needs, the next step is to set specific, measurable, achievable, relevant, and time-bound (SMART) goals. For example, instead of setting a vague goal like "I want to eat healthier," consider specifying, "I will incorporate at least three servings of fruits and vegetables into my meals each day." This clarity will make it easier to track your progress and stay motivated.

Setting SMART goals means breaking down larger objectives into smaller, manageable steps. If your goal is to exercise more regularly, you might start with a commitment to walk for 20 minutes three times a week. As you become more comfortable, you can gradually increase the duration and intensity of your workouts. This approach prevents feelings of overwhelm and helps you build confidence in your ability to achieve your wellness goals.

Additionally, it's important to align your goals with your values and aspirations. Consider what wellness means to you personally. Does it involve physical fitness, emotional resilience, social connections, or a combination of these elements? Reflecting on your values will ensure that your wellness plan resonates with who you are and what you want to achieve in life.

Tracking Progress and Maintaining Health Habits

Tracking your progress is a vital component of any wellness plan. Regularly reviewing your goals allows you to see how far you've come and identify areas for improvement. Keeping a journal or using a mobile app can be effective tools for tracking your health habits. You might note your daily food intake, exercise routines, and stress levels, or reflect on your emotional well-being.

When tracking your progress, it can be helpful to create a chart or a checklist. For instance, if you aim to incorporate more physical activity into your routine, you might create a weekly exercise log where you record the type of activity, duration, and how you felt afterward. Over time, this data can help you identify trends in your activity levels and how they correlate with your overall well-being.

Establishing a routine can significantly contribute to maintaining health habits. Choose specific days and times for activities like exercise, meal prep, and self-care. Treat these appointments with the same importance as you would academic commitments. By scheduling wellness practices into your weekly routine, you create a structure that encourages consistency.

For instance, if you know that you have a free hour on Wednesdays and Fridays, you could block off that time for a workout or a yoga class. This commitment not only helps you prioritize your health but also makes it easier to avoid the temptation of skipping out on self-care due to academic stress.

Accountability is another powerful motivator. Consider sharing your wellness goals with a trusted friend or family member who can provide encouragement and support. Regular check-ins with this accountability partner can help you stay on track and celebrate your successes together. Alternatively, you might find a wellness buddy—a fellow student with similar health goals—who can join you in workouts or study sessions focused on self-care.

Adjusting Your Wellness Plan as Life Changes

Life is full of transitions, especially during college. From changing majors and moving to new living situations to entering the workforce, these shifts can impact your wellness plan. It's essential to remain flexible and adjust your plan as needed to accommodate life changes.

If you find that your current exercise routine no longer fits your schedule or that you need to adjust your dietary goals due to financial constraints, don't hesitate to modify your approach. The key is to remain adaptable and recognize that setbacks are a natural part of the journey.

For example, if you've experienced a significant change, like a new job or a demanding course load, your previous wellness practices might need reevaluation. If you were exercising five times a week but now struggle to find time, it may be more beneficial to focus on shorter, more efficient workouts or find alternative ways to stay active, such as taking the stairs instead of the elevator or incorporating quick stretching breaks during study sessions.

Regularly revisiting your goals and assessing their relevance will help ensure that your wellness plan continues to serve your evolving needs. Reflect on what's working, what's not, and where you can make adjustments to better align your practices with your current situation.

Integrating Wellness Practices into Your Post-College Life

As you approach graduation and transition into the next phase of your life, it's crucial to consider how you will maintain your wellness practices beyond college. The skills and habits you develop now will lay the foundation for a healthy lifestyle as you navigate the demands of the professional world.

Begin by identifying which wellness practices have been most beneficial during your college years. Are there specific exercise routines, stress management techniques, or social activities that you want to carry forward? Create a plan for integrating these practices into your post-college life. Consider setting aside dedicated time each week for exercise, continuing mindfulness practices, or maintaining social connections that nourish you.

Transitioning from college to the workforce can be a significant adjustment, often accompanied by new stresses and responsibilities. To help mitigate these challenges, look for opportunities to engage with wellness communities outside of college. Many cities offer yoga studios, fitness classes, and wellness workshops that can help you continue your journey toward holistic health. Networking with like-minded individuals in these settings can also foster social connections and support your commitment to maintaining a balanced lifestyle.

Additionally, consider how your career choices may impact your wellness. Some jobs may demand long hours, while others may offer more flexibility. Reflect on your values and how they align with your career aspirations. If maintaining work-life balance is essential to you, seek opportunities that promote this principle.

Staying Committed to a Lifelong Journey of Health and Balance

The journey of health and wellness is ongoing, and staying committed to this path requires intentionality and reflection. Regularly revisit your goals, assess your progress, and celebrate your achievements, no matter how small they may seem. Acknowledging your successes reinforces your commitment and motivates you to continue prioritizing your health.

To support your commitment, consider creating a vision board or a wellness manifesto—a visual representation of your health goals and values. This can serve as a daily reminder of what you're working toward and help you stay inspired. Display your board in a place where you'll see it regularly, like your bedroom or workspace.

It's also essential to practice self-compassion as you navigate your wellness journey. There will be times when you encounter setbacks or challenges, and that's okay. Instead of being critical of yourself, recognize that these moments are opportunities for growth and learning. Embrace the idea that wellness is not a destination but a lifelong journey filled with ups and downs.

Engaging in lifelong learning about health and wellness can further support your commitment. Stay curious about new wellness practices, nutrition trends, and mental health strategies. Reading books, attending workshops, or following credible wellness experts on social media can provide valuable insights and inspire you to explore new avenues for health.

Consider also creating a list of resources that you can return to as you navigate different stages of life. This list could include books, podcasts, websites, and local services related to nutrition, fitness, mental health, and self-care. Having these resources at your fingertips can empower you to make informed decisions about your health and wellness.

In conclusion, creating a personal wellness plan is an empowering step toward taking control of your health and well-being during college and beyond. By assessing your needs, setting specific goals, tracking your progress, and remaining adaptable, you can establish a sustainable approach to wellness. Integrating your practices into post-college life and committing to lifelong health will ensure you continue to thrive in all areas of your life.

Conclusion: Your Path to a Healthier, Happier College Experience

As you reach the end of this book, it's essential to take a moment to reflect on your growth and achievements throughout your college journey. Navigating the demands of academia while prioritizing your health is no small feat. By embracing holistic health principles, you have taken significant strides toward creating a balanced, fulfilling college experience. This journey has empowered you to cultivate habits that nourish your mind, body, and spirit, laying a strong foundation for your future.

Reflecting on Your Growth and Achievements

Consider the progress you have made in various aspects of your life. From managing stress to improving your nutrition and maintaining healthy relationships, each step you've taken contributes to a healthier, more resilient you. Acknowledge the challenges you've overcome, whether it be implementing new study strategies, finding time for exercise, or fostering connections with supportive peers. Each achievement, big or small, deserves recognition, as it reflects your commitment to prioritizing your well-being amidst the complexities of college life.

Reflecting on your experiences can also provide valuable insights into your personal growth. What strategies worked well for you? What challenges did you face, and how did you overcome them? Taking the time to write down these reflections can serve as a powerful reminder of your resilience and determination. Consider creating a journal where you document your health journey, noting the positive changes you have made and the impact they have had on your life.

Embracing Self-Care as an Ongoing Practice

Self-care is not a one-time effort but an ongoing practice that requires attention and dedication. As you continue your journey beyond college, remember that prioritizing your well-being is crucial for sustaining your mental, emotional, and physical health. Incorporating self-care rituals into your daily routine will empower you to navigate life's challenges with grace and resilience. Whether it's setting aside time for mindfulness, engaging in physical activity, or simply allowing yourself moments of rest, these practices will enhance your overall quality of life.

Recognizing the importance of self-care can be a game-changer in your post-college life. In a world that often emphasizes productivity and achievement, it's vital to counterbalance those pressures with activities that rejuvenate your spirit. Consider establishing a self-care schedule that includes various activities, such as yoga, meditation, reading, or engaging in hobbies that bring you joy.

Self-care also extends to your mental health. Seek out activities that promote relaxation and reduce stress. This may include mindfulness practices, breathing exercises, or even therapy sessions. Prioritizing mental health is a sign of strength and a crucial component of holistic health.

Words of Encouragement for the Journey Ahead

The transition from college to the next chapter of your life can be both exciting and daunting. As you embark on this new journey, remember that it is perfectly normal to feel a mix of anticipation and uncertainty as you venture into new territories. Embrace this journey as an opportunity for growth, learning, and self-discovery. Carry the lessons you've learned about holistic health with you, and don't hesitate to adapt your practices as your circumstances evolve.

As you face new challenges, remind yourself that you possess the tools and resilience to navigate whatever comes your way. Your commitment to your health and well-being is an invaluable asset that will serve you well in the years to come. Surround yourself with a supportive community, seek resources when needed, and be open to change and growth.

Life beyond college may come with its own set of challenges, such as entering the workforce or adapting to a new living environment. Keep in mind that the habits you have built during your time in college can help you navigate these transitions. Embrace flexibility and remember that change is a natural part of life. Be patient with yourself as you adjust to new responsibilities and routines.

Resources for Continued Learning and Wellness

To further support your journey toward holistic health, consider seeking out additional resources. Numerous books, podcasts, online courses, and wellness communities are dedicated to personal growth and self-care. Engaging with these resources can deepen your understanding of health and provide inspiration as you explore new practices.

Look for local workshops or seminars focused on nutrition, fitness, mindfulness, and mental health. Connecting with professionals in these fields can offer valuable insights and practical tools for maintaining your well-being.

Additionally, many colleges and universities offer wellness programs that can provide ongoing support and education.

Online platforms can also be an excellent resource for continued learning. Websites, apps, and social media channels dedicated to holistic health and wellness can provide daily tips, recipes, and encouragement to keep you motivated. Consider joining online forums or support groups where you can connect with others who share your commitment to health.

Celebrating Your Commitment to Holistic Health

Finally, celebrate your commitment to holistic health. Acknowledge the effort you've put into creating a healthier, happier college experience, and recognize the positive impact these changes have made on your life. Whether it's treating yourself to a special day of self-care, sharing your journey with friends, or simply taking a moment to reflect in gratitude, honoring your dedication to wellness is an essential part of the process.

Consider hosting a wellness celebration with friends or fellow students who have been part of your journey. Share your experiences, lessons learned, and successes. This not only reinforces your commitment to holistic health but also fosters a sense of community and support among your peers.

As you continue to grow, keep in mind that your commitment to health is a lifelong journey. Each step you take contributes to a more vibrant, balanced life. Embrace the small victories along the way, and don't shy away from celebrating your achievements, no matter how minor they may seem.

As you move forward, carry the principles of holistic health with you. You have the power to shape your future and create a life that aligns with your values and aspirations. Embrace each day as an opportunity to prioritize your health and well-being, and remember that you are capable of achieving balance and fulfillment in every aspect of your life.

Your Holistic Journey Continues

Your journey toward holistic health does not end with the completion of this book. Rather, it serves as a stepping stone for a lifetime of learning and growth. Continue to seek knowledge and inspiration as you explore new avenues for health and wellness. Remember that each phase of your life may require different strategies and approaches, and it's perfectly okay to evolve your practices over time.

Engage with mentors, attend workshops, and read widely to expand your understanding of holistic health. Your journey may take you through various stages—each providing its own unique lessons and insights. Embrace the process and remain curious about how you can continue to enhance your well-being.

In conclusion, thank you for joining me on this journey toward holistic health. May you continue to thrive in your college experience and beyond, empowered by the knowledge and practices you've cultivated along the way. Your path to a healthier, happier life is just beginning, and I have no doubt that you will navigate it with grace and determination. You possess the tools to create a fulfilling and balanced life, and I wish you all the best on your journey ahead.

Glossary of Terms

Balance: The state of equilibrium in various aspects of life, including physical, emotional, and social well-being. Striving for balance helps to reduce stress and enhance overall health.

Burnout: A state of emotional, physical, and mental exhaustion caused by prolonged stress, often resulting from excessive demands in academic or personal life.

Coping Mechanisms: Strategies and techniques that individuals use to manage stress, anxiety, and difficult emotions. Healthy coping mechanisms can promote resilience and emotional well-being.

Emotional Well-being: The ability to understand, manage, and express emotions effectively, contributing to a person's overall mental health and quality of life.

Holistic Health: An approach to health that considers the whole person—mind, body, and spirit—rather than focusing solely on physical symptoms. Holistic health emphasizes the interconnectedness of various aspects of well-being.

Mindfulness: A mental practice that involves focusing on the present moment without judgment. Mindfulness can reduce stress, enhance emotional regulation, and promote mental clarity.

Nutrition: The study of how food affects health and well-being. Proper nutrition is essential for physical health, cognitive function, and emotional balance, especially in high-stress environments like college.

Resilience: The ability to adapt to challenges, stress, and adversity while maintaining a positive outlook. Resilience is a key component of mental health and well-being.

Self-Care: Activities and practices that individuals engage in to promote their own physical, emotional, and mental health. Self-care is essential for maintaining balance and preventing burnout.

Social Support: The emotional, informational, and practical assistance provided by family, friends, and community. Strong social support networks can enhance resilience and reduce feelings of isolation.

Stress Management: Techniques and strategies used to control stress levels and reduce the impact of stress on health. Effective stress management can lead to improved well-being and academic performance.

Wellness Plan: A personalized strategy for maintaining and improving health, encompassing physical, mental, and emotional components. A wellness plan can help individuals set goals and track progress toward better health.

Did You Enjoy This Book?

Dear Reader,

I hope this message finds you well. I wanted to take a moment to express my sincere gratitude for choosing to read ***Holistic Health for College Students: Practical Tips for Staying Healthy and Balanced in College***. It means the world to me that you've invested your time and trust in my work.

If you found *Holistic Health for College Students* enjoyable and valuable, I would be immensely grateful if you could spare a few moments to leave a review on Amazon, Goodreads, etc. Your feedback not only helps other readers discover the book but also provides valuable insights for me as an author.

Whether it's a brief comment about what you liked most, how the book impacted you, or simply your overall impression, your review would make a significant difference. Your honest opinion is invaluable in helping me grow as a writer and in reaching more readers.

Thank you so much for your support and for being a part of this journey with me. Your reviews truly mean the world to me.

Warmest regards,

Angelina Sorenson

Three Isles Publishing

About the Author

Angelina Sorenson is a wellness advocate, speaker, and author dedicated to helping young adults thrive in every aspect of their lives. With a background in holistic health and a passion for empowering college students, Angelina combines practical knowledge with a deep understanding of the unique challenges young adults face. She has spent over a decade developing wellness workshops for students, focusing on stress management, balanced living, and self-care practices.

Angelina's approach emphasizes the importance of mental, emotional, and physical well-being, offering practical, accessible strategies that fit seamlessly into busy college life. Her work has helped countless students build resilience, create positive habits, and stay grounded in their values.

When she's not writing or working with students, Angelina enjoys hiking, exploring new cuisines, and practicing mindfulness meditation. Through her books and workshops, Angelina continues to share her insights, aiming to inspire young adults to live healthier, more balanced lives.